100 Immune System Boosting Meal and Juice Recipes:

Strengthen Your Immune System Using Natural Foods

By

Joe Correa CSN

COPYRIGHT

ACKNOWLEDGEMENTS

This book is dedicated to my friends and family that have had mild or serious illnesses so that you may find a solution and make the necessary changes in your life.

100 Immune System Boosting Meal and Juice Recipes:

Strengthen Your Immune System Using Natural Foods

By

Joe Correa CSN

CONTENTS

ABOUT THE AUTHOR

After years of Research, I honestly believe in the positive effects that proper nutrition can have over the body and mind. My knowledge and experience has helped me live healthier throughout the years and which I have shared with family and friends. The more you know about eating and drinking healthier, the sooner you will want to change your life and eating habits.

Nutrition is a key part in the process of being healthy and living longer so get started today. The first step is the most important and the most significant.

INTRODUCTION

100 Immune System Boosting Meal and Juice Recipes: Strengthen Your Immune System Using Natural Foods

By Joe Correa CSN

The main reason doctors say people get sick is because of a weak immune system. Having a weak immune system makes it much harder for your body to fight infections, diseases, and any other harmful substances. Exercise and diet are the fastest way to strengthen your immune system. Fruits that are high in vitamin C like strawberries, blueberries, lemon, passion fruit, tangerines, grapefruit, etc.

By including these fruits in your diet on a normal basis you will drastically change your body's capacity to defend itself. The recipes in this book have a variety of ingredients that are vitamin packed and are high in vitamin C which will help you achieve your goal to strengthen your immune system and fight off harmful diseases and infections. Honey and agave syrup are excellent choices when it comes to sweetening your food since they offer a natural source of sugar that your body and quickly absorb. Other potent ingredients we have included are: oats, beetroot, lactose free milk, cereals, peanuts, raisins, pecans, sesame, and linseed, just to name a few.

Make the decision to help your body by giving it what it needs to defend itself. When it comes to getting healthy and staying healthy there's only one choice, eating right!

COMMITMENT

In order to improve my condition, I *(your name)*, commit to eating more of these foods on a daily basis and to exercise at least 30 minutes daily:

- Berries (especially blueberries), peaches, cherries, apples, apricots, oranges, lemon juice, grapefruit, tangerines, mandarins, pears, etc.
- Broccoli, spinach, collard greens, sweet potatoes, avocado, artichoke, baby corn, carrots, celery, cauliflower, onions, etc.
- Whole grains, steel-cut oats, oatmeal, quinoa, barley, etc.
- Black beans, red bean beans, garbanzo beans, lentils, etc.
- Nuts and seeds including: walnuts, cashews, flaxseeds, sesame seeds, etc.
- Fish
- 8 – 10 glasses of water

Sign here

X_____

100 IMMUNE SYSTEM BOOSTING MEAL AND JUICE RECIPES: STRENGTHEN YOUR IMMUNE SYSTEM USING NATURAL FOODS

JUICES

1.   Camu Camu shake (6 people)

Ingredients:

- 3 spoons of camu camu powder or 1 cup of camu camu cut in cubes
- 1 cup of water
- 2 cups of chopped papaya
- 2 cups of strawberries
- 1/2 cup of ice cubes
- 2 spoons of natural honey

Procedure: In a blender mix the camu camu, strawberries and the ice. Add the honey and mix. Serve in 4 glasses. You can accompany this powerful shake with oat pancakes to make the perfect combination.

Nutritional facts: Energy 100 kcal, total fat 0 g, cholesterol 0 mg, carbohydrates 22 g and fiber 3 g.

2.   Tropical shake (4 people)

Ingredients:

- 3 cups of chopped papaya

- 1 cup of chopped mango

- 1 cup of chopped strawberries

- 2 cups of natural yogurt

- 1 ½ cups of chopped pineapple

- 1 cup of ice cubes

- 2 spoons of linseed powder

Procedure: In a blender mix all the ingredients until you get a creamy look. In case you may need something to dissolve it if the juice is too dense you can add half a cup of water. Serve immediately.

Nutritional facts: Energy 194 kcal, total fat 4 g, cholesterol 7 mg, carbohydrates 35 g and fiber 5 g.

3.   Beetroot delights (2 people)

Ingredients:

- 1 cup of apples cut in cubes without skin
- 1/2 cup of beetroot cut in cubes
- 4 chopped carrots without skin
- 1 cup of green tee
- 2 spoons of natural honey

Procedure: Grate the carrots, beetroot, and apples. In a blender mix the grated carrots, beetroot, apples and tee. Add honey to make it sweet. Serve in tall glasses.

Nutritional facts: Energy 252 kcal, total fat 10 g, cholesterol 8 mg, carbohydrates 44 g and fiber 5 g.

4.   Energetic juice (4 people)

Ingredients:

- 1 cup of natural yogurt
- 1 banana
- 1 cup of orange juice
- 8 strawberries

Procedure: Cut the leaves off the strawberries and wash. In a blender mix all the ingredients until you get a creamy look. Serve and enjoy.

Nutritional facts: Energy 213 kcal, total fat 0 g, cholesterol 0 mg, carbohydrates 38 g and fiber 3 g.

5. Carrots extract (2 people)

Ingredients:

- 8 carrots without skin
- 2 spoons of ginger powder
- 1 spoon of linseed powder
- 1 cup of water

Procedure: Grate the carrots. In a blender mix the grated carrots, ginger, linseed and water. Add honey if needed. Serve in tall glasses. This is a great juice to have in the morning or afternoon and can be accompanied with an omelet.

Nutritional facts: Energy 221 kcal, total fat 8 g, cholesterol 11 mg, carbohydrates 64 g and fiber 5 g.

6.   Vitamin C booster (3 people)

Ingredients:

- 1/2 banana

- 1/2 cup of strawberries

- 1/2 cup of orange juice

- 2 mints leaves

- 1 cup of green tee

Procedure: In a blender mix all the ingredients until you get a creamy look. In case you may need something to dissolve it if the juice is too dense you can always add a half cup of water. Serve immediately.

Nutritional facts: Energy 232 kcal, total fat 10 g, cholesterol 19 mg, carbohydrates 46 g and fiber 4 g.

7.   Coconut - lemon (5 people)

Ingredients:

- 3/4 cup of lemon juice

- 4 spoons of natural honey

- 1 cup of coconut cream

- 6 ice cubes

- 1/2 cup of coconut in slices

- 1 grated lemon

Procedure: In a blender mix 1 liter of water, lemon juice, honey, coconut cream and ice. Serve and decorate with the coconut and the grated lemon.

Nutritional facts: Energy 234 kcal, total fat 9 g, cholesterol 16 mg, carbohydrates 54 g and fiber 4 g.

8.   Mango delights (4 people)

Ingredients:

- 2 cups of strawberries cut in slices

- 2 bananas cut in slice

- 1 mango cut in squares

- 1 cup of natural yogurt

- 1 spoons of natural honey

- 1 cup of ice cubes

Procedure: In a blender mix the strawberries, bananas, and mango. Gradually add the yogurt until you get a creamy look. Pour a half cup to a cup of water if necessary. Add the ice cubes and mix again. Serve immediately.

Nutritional facts: Energy 256 kcal, total fat 4 g, cholesterol 8 mg, carbohydrates 68 g and fiber 4 g.

9.   Oats and sesame shake (2 people)

Ingredients:

- 1 cup of almonds milk

- 1 spoon of wheat germ

- 2 spoons of toasted oats

- 1 spoon of toasted sesame seeds

- 1 spoon of almonds

- 2 spoon of natural honey

Procedure: In a blender pour the glass of almond milk; then add the wheat germ, oats, sesame seeds, and almonds. Dress with honey. Serve immediately.

Nutritional facts: Energy 259 kcal, total fat 9 g, cholesterol 14 mg, carbohydrates 32 g and fiber 7 g.

10. Quick beetroot juice (1 person)

Ingredients:

- 1 beetroot
- 1 carrot
- 1 glass of water

Procedure: Peel, cut and put the beetroot into the mixer. Cut the carrot in squares and add to the mixer. Add a glass of water and shake until you get a creamy look.

Nutritional facts: Energy 254 kcal, total fat 0 g, cholesterol 0 mg, carbohydrates 56 g and fiber 6 g.

11.   Cranberry mix (1 person)

Ingredients:

- 1 cup of organic cranberry juice (250 ml)
- 1/2 cup of water
- 1 spoon of olive oil
- 2 spoons of natural honey

Procedure: Take all the ingredients and put them in the blender and mix until you get a consistent look. This a strong mix of ingredients that should be consumed early in the morning.

Nutritional facts: Energy 198 kcal, total fat 1 g, cholesterol 1 mg, carbohydrates 43 g and fiber 4 g.

12.   Acid parsley juice (2 people)

Ingredients:

- 1 cup of fresh parsley
- 1 green apple
- juice of ½ lemon
- 1/2 spoon of grated ginger
- 1 cup of water

Procedure: Chop the parsley and apple. Introduce all the ingredients to the blender and mix. Strain the juice. Serve immediately. Drink before breakfast if possible.

Nutritional facts: Energy 222 kcal, total fat 4 g, cholesterol 0 mg, carbohydrates 57 g and fiber 5 g.

13.　Fennel and lettuce juice (2 people)

Ingredients:

- 9 lettuce leaves (avoid the Iceberg variety which does not content so many nutrients)
- 1 slice of fresh fennel root (5 cm)
- 1 spoon of natural honey
- 1/2 cup of water

Procedure: Wash and clean the lettuce leaves and then finely chop them. Put all the ingredients in a blender and mix. Strain the juice and serve in tall glasses.

Nutritional facts: Energy 176 kcal, total fat 0 g, cholesterol 0 mg, carbohydrates 57 g and fiber 4 g.

14.   Parsley shake (2 people)

Ingredients:

- 1/2 cucumber

- 100 gr of parsley

- 1/2 lactose free milk

- 1/2 cup of water

- 2 spoons of natural honey

Procedure: Wash the cucumber and parsley. Cut the cucumber in slices and chop the parsley. Put everything in the blender and mix. Strain and serve immediately.

Nutritional facts: Energy 176 kcal, total fat 6 g, cholesterol 7 mg, carbohydrates 35 g and fiber 2 g.

15.   Refreshing juice (2 people)

Ingredients:

- 250 g of strawberries

- 2 pineapple slices

- 1 cup of water

Procedure: Wash the strawberries and take the green leaves out. Cut the pineapple slices in half and make sure you take the skin out. Chop the strawberries and pineapple into small pieces. Put everything in a blender and mix until you get a creamy look. Strain and when done.

Nutritional facts: Energy 189 kcal, total fat 0 g, cholesterol 0 mg, carbohydrates 22 g and fiber 2 g.

16.   Grape juice (2 people)

Ingredients:

- 250 g of red grapes
- 1 cup of water
- 1/2 spoon of mint
- 2 spoons of honey

Procedure: Wash the grapes. Peel the grapes and then cut by the half to take the seeds out. Put everything in a blender and mix. Serve immediately.

Nutritional facts: Energy 165 kcal, total fat 0 g, cholesterol 0 mg, carbohydrates 36 g and fiber 4 g.

17. Good morning refresher (2 people)

Ingredients:

- 4 cups of fresh watermelon cut in cubes

- 4 spoons of lemon juice

- 1/2 cup of water

- 2 spoons of honey

Procedure: Mix everything in a blender until you get a creamy look. Dress with honey and mix again. Serve in large glasses.

Nutritional facts: Energy 175 kcal, total fat 0 g, cholesterol 0 mg, carbohydrates 28 g and fiber 3 g.

18.   Radish and celery juice (2 people)

Ingredients:

- 3 cups of radishes

- 3 celery steams

- 1 cup of water

Procedure: Wash the radishes and celery. Peel the radish and cut in thin slices. Chop the celery. Add water and blend. Strain and serve immediately.

Nutritional facts: Energy 176 kcal, total fat 0 g, cholesterol 0 mg, carbohydrates 31 g and fiber 2 g.

19. Asparagus delights (2 people)

Ingredients:

- 2 asparagus

- 1 apple

- 1 broccoli steam

- 2 carrots

- 1 cup of water

- 2 spoons of natural honey

Procedure: Mix everything in a blender and add water progressively according to the consistence you want to get. Once you have a creamy look you are ready to strain the juice. Serve and enjoy.

Nutritional facts: Energy 258 kcal, total fat 3 g, cholesterol 3 mg, carbohydrates 43 g and fiber 6 g.

20. Acai-berry mix juice (2 people)

Ingredients:

- 1/2 cup of orange juice
- 1 banana cut in slices
- 1 mango cut in slices
- 1 cup of pulp of acai berries
- 1 cup of water
- 2 spoons of natural honey

Procedure: Mix everything in a blender and add water progressively according to the consistency you want to get. Once you have a creamy look serve and enjoy.

Nutritional facts: Energy 276 kcal, total fat 10 g, cholesterol 9 mg, carbohydrates 64 g and fiber 5 g.

21. Pumpkin and coco mix (2 people)

Ingredients:

- 1 glass of water

- 1 glass of coconut juice

- 1/2 cup of cooked pumpkin

- 1 spoon of honey

Procedure: In a blender mix the coconut, water and pumpkin for a few minutes until you get a creamy look. Pour the juice in tall glasses and add the honey and mix again. Enjoy.

Nutritional facts: Energy 198 kcal, total fat 2 g, cholesterol 6 mg, carbohydrates 66 g and fiber 4 g.

22.   Blueberry shake (2 people)

Ingredients:

- 1/4 cup of lactose free milk

- 3/4 cup of natural yogurt

- 1 cup of blueberries

- 1 spoon of linseed powder

Procedure: Wash the blueberries. Mix everything in a blender until you get a creamy look. Add water progressively if you want a more liquid mixture. Serve immediately.

Nutritional facts: Energy 198 kcal, total fat 11 g, cholesterol 21 mg, carbohydrates 54 g and fiber 2 g.

23.   Orange milkshake (2 people)

Ingredients:

- 1 cup of orange juice

- 1/2 cup of water

- 1/2 spoon of vanilla essence

- 1/2 cup of lactose free milk

- 2 spoons of honey

- 5 ice cubes

Procedure: Mix everything in a blender until you get a creamy look. Add water progressively if you want a more liquid mixture. Serve in large glasses.

Nutritional facts: Energy 212 kcal, total fat 3 g, cholesterol 6 mg, carbohydrates 48 g and fiber 2 g.

24.   Popeye shake (2 people)

Ingredients:

- 1 ½ cup of green tee
- 1 cup of spinach
- 1/2 cup of water
- 1 apple
- 1 pear
- 1 spoon of honey
- 1 spoon of lime

Procedure: Wash the spinach, apple and pear. Peel the apple and pear. Chop the spinach, apple and pear. Mix everything in a blender until you get a creamy look. Add water progressively if you want a more liquid mixture. Serve and enjoy.

Nutritional facts: Energy 232 kcal, total fat 3 g, cholesterol 4 mg, carbohydrates 46 g and fiber 4 g.

25.   Carrot booster (2 people)

Ingredients:

- 1 cup of pineapple cut in cubes
- 1 cup of grated carrots
- 1/2 cup of strawberries
- 1 cup of water
- juice from 2 oranges

Procedure: Mix everything in a blender until you get a creamy look. Add the water progressively if you want a more liquid mixture. Serve and enjoy.

Nutritional facts: Energy 178 kcal, total fat 6 g, cholesterol 6 mg, carbohydrates 54 g and fiber 4 g.

26.   Banana-strength shake (2 people)

Ingredients:

- 3/4 cup of milk
- 1/4 cup of granola
- 1 banana
- 1 cup of ice cubes
- 2 spoons of linseed powder

Procedure: Mix everything in a blender until you get a creamy look. Add water progressively if you want a more liquid mixture. Serve immediately.

Nutritional facts: Energy 276 kcal, total fat 7 g, cholesterol 7 mg, carbohydrates 32 g and fiber 7 g.

27.   Spinach mix (2 people)

Ingredients:

- 1 banana
- 1/2 cup of chopped spinach
- 1 spoon of peanut butter
- 1 ½ cup of lactose free milk
- 1 spoon of linseed powder
- 1 spoon of sesame seeds

Procedure: Mix everything in a blender until you get a creamy look. Add water progressively if you want a more liquid mixture. Serve in large glasses. Decorate with sesame seeds and enjoy.

Nutritional facts: Energy 230 kcal, total fat 9 g, cholesterol 9 mg, carbohydrates 23 g and fiber 7 g.

28.   Kale power juice (2 people)

Ingredients:

- 1 cup of fresh kale

- 1 cup of almond milk

- 1 cup of blueberries

- 1/2 banana

- 1 spoon of almond butter

- 2 spoon of instant oats

Procedure: Mix everything in a blender until you get a creamy look. Add water progressively if you want a more liquid mixture. Serve immediately.

Nutritional facts: Energy 256 kcal, total fat 9 g, cholesterol 8 mg, carbohydrates 25 g and fiber 12 g.

29.   Almonds and peanuts mix (2 people)

Ingredients:

- 2 cups of coconut water

- 6 almonds

- 1 spoon of vanilla essence

- 1 spoon of cinnamon

- 1 cup of chopped apple

- 1/2 cup of peanuts

Procedure: Mix everything in a blender until you get a creamy look. Add water progressively if you want a more liquid mixture. Serve in tall glasses.

Nutritional facts: Energy 218 kcal, total fat 6 g, cholesterol 5 mg, carbohydrates 46 g and fiber 4 g.

30.   Blueberry booster (2 people)

Ingredients:

- 1 banana

- 1 cup of blueberries

- 1/3 cup of instant oats

- 1 cup of lactose free milk

Procedure: Put the banana and blueberries in the fridge for 10 minutes. Mix everything in a blender until you get a creamy look. Add water progressively if you want a more liquid mixture. Serve immediately.

Nutritional facts: Energy 214 kcal, total fat 4 g, cholesterol 0 mg, carbohydrates 64 g and fiber 4 g.

31.   Strawberry delights (2 people)

Ingredients:

- 1/2 cup of raspberries

- 1 cup of strawberries

- 1 cup of mango

- 1 cup of water

- 2 spoons of honey

Procedure: Put the fruits into the fridge for 10 minutes. Mix everything in a blender until you get a creamy look. Add water progressively if you want a more liquid mixture. Serve and enjoy.

Nutritional facts: Energy 214 kcal, total fat 5 g, cholesterol 0 mg, carbohydrates 48 g and fiber 4 g.

32.   Blueberry delights (2 people)

Ingredients:

- 1 cup of raspberries
- 1 cup of blueberries
- 1 cup of strawberries
- 1/2 cup of natural yogurt
- 1/2 cup of green tee

Procedure: Mix everything in a blender until you get a creamy look. Add the water progressively if you want a more liquid mixture. Serve in tall glasses.

Nutritional facts: Energy 198 kcal, total fat 4 g, cholesterol 5 mg, carbohydrates 38 g and fiber 4 g.

33.   Kiwi and strawberry mix (2 people)

Ingredients:

- 2 chopped kiwis

- 1/2 cup of chopped peaches

- 1 ½ cup of strawberries

- 1 cup of water

- 2 spoons of honey

Procedure: Mix everything in a blender until you get a creamy look. Add water progressively if you want a more liquid mixture. Serve immediately.

Nutritional facts: Energy 213 kcal, total fat 2 g, cholesterol 0 mg, carbohydrates 45 g and fiber 5 g.

34.   Straw-nana juice (2 people)

Ingredients:

- 1/2 cup of chopped pineapple

- 1 banana

- 1/2 cup of mango cut in slices

- 1 cup of strawberries

- 1 cup of lactose free milk

Procedure: Mix everything in a blender until you get a creamy look. Add water progressively if you want a more liquid mixture. Serve and enjoy.

Nutritional facts: Energy 215 kcal, total fat 3 g, cholesterol 6 mg, carbohydrates 53 g and fiber 5 g.

35.   Assorted delights (2 people)

Ingredients:

- 1 chopped kiwi

- 1 ½ cups of watermelon cut in cubes

- 1 ½ cups of red grapes

- 1 cup of lactose free milk

- 1 spoon of vanilla essence

- 1 spoon of honey

Procedure: Peel the grapes and then cut by the half. Take all the seeds out if they have them. Mix everything in a blender until you get a creamy look. Add water progressively if you want a more liquid texture. Serve immediately.

Nutritional facts: Energy 245 kcal, total fat 6 g, cholesterol 7 mg, carbohydrates 48 g and fiber 5 g.

36.   Blue spinach (2 people)

Ingredients:

- 1 cup of blueberries

- 1 cup of peaches

- 1 cup of chopped spinach

- 1/2 cup of natural yogurt

- 1/2 cup of green tee

Procedure: Put everything in a blender and mix until you get a consistent look. Add water progressively if you want a more liquid mixture. Serve in tall glasses.

Nutritional facts: Energy 238 kcal, total fat 3 g, cholesterol 7 mg, carbohydrates 54 g and fiber 5 g.

37. Strawberry smoothie (2 people)

Ingredients:

- 1/2 cup of instant oats

- 1 cup of banana

- 14 frozen strawberries

- 1 cup of lactose free milk

- 2 spoons of honey

- 1 spoon of vanilla essence

Procedure: Mix everything in a blender until you get a creamy look. Add water progressively if you want a more liquid mixture. Serve in tall glasses.

Nutritional facts: Energy 267 kcal, total fat 5 g, cholesterol 9 mg, carbohydrates 58 g and fiber 6 g.

38.   Green delicate (2 people)

Ingredients:

- 1/2 cup of water

- 1 spoon of lime juice

- 2 chopped kiwis

- 1 chopped pear

- 2 spoons of honey

- 1/2 cup of ice cubes

Procedure: Mix everything in a blender until you get a creamy look. Add water progressively if you want a more liquid mixture. Serve immediately.

Nutritional facts: Energy 221 kcal, total fat 2 g, cholesterol 0 mg, carbohydrates 64 g and fiber 5 g.

39.   Mango delights (2 people)

Ingredients:

- 2 mangos cut in slices

- 1 cup of natural yogurt

- 1 cup of water

- 1 banana

- 2 spoons of lemon juice

- 1 spoon of vanilla essence

Procedure: Mix everything in a blender until you get a creamy look. Add water progressively if you want a more liquid mixture. Serve and enjoy.

Nutritional facts: Energy 198 kcal, total fat 3 g, cholesterol 7 mg, carbohydrates 46 g and fiber 4 g.

40. Pineapple smoothie (2 people)

Ingredients:

- 2 cups of chopped pineapple
- 1 banana cut in cubes
- 1/2 cup of natural yogurt
- 1/2 cup of water
- 1/2 cup of ice cubes
- 2 spoons of natural honey

Procedure: Mix everything in a blender until you get a creamy look. Add water progressively if you want a more liquid mixture. Serve immediately.

Nutritional facts: Energy 236 kcal, total fat 3 g, cholesterol 7 mg, carbohydrates 58 g and fiber 6 g.

41. Cranberry smoothie (2 people)

Ingredients:

- 1 cup of natural yogurt
- 1/2 cup of cranberries
- 1 cup of bananas cut in slices
- 2 oranges cut in cubes
- 1/2 cup of water
- 3 spoons of honey

Procedure: Mix everything in a blender until you get a creamy look. Add water progressively if you want a more liquid mixture. Serve immediately.

Nutritional facts: Energy 232 kcal, total fat 3 g, cholesterol 7 mg, carbohydrates 62 g and fiber 6 g.

42.   Berries mix (2 people)

Ingredients:

- 2 cups of strawberries

- 1/2 cup of blackberries

- 1/2 cup of blueberries

- 1 cup of chopped apricot

- 1 cup of water

- 3 spoons of honey

Procedure: Put all the fruits into the fridge for 10 minutes. Mix everything in a blender until you get a creamy look. Add water progressively if you want a more liquid mixture. Serve in tall glasses.

Nutritional facts: Energy 222 kcal, total fat 2 g, cholesterol 0 mg, carbohydrates 58 g and fiber 6 g.

43.   Raspberry-mint juice (2 people)

Ingredients:

- 2 cups of raspberries cut in cubes
- 1 cup of water
- 1 cup of lactose free milk
- 1 cup of chopped mango
- 1/2 cup of chopped mint leaves
- 1 spoon of lemon juice
- 1 pinch of salt
- 1/2 cup of ice cubes

Procedure: Take the fruits to the fridge for 10 minutes. Mix everything in a blender until you get a creamy look. Add water progressively if you want a more liquid mixture. Serve immediately.

Nutritional facts: Energy 243 kcal, total fat 3 g, cholesterol 7 mg, carbohydrates 54 g and fiber 7 g.

44. Almond and sesame juice (2 people)

Ingredients:

- 1/2 cup of peanuts
- 1/2 cup of cherries
- 1 banana
- 1 spoon of sesame seeds
- 1 cup of almond milk
- 1 spoon of grated almonds

Procedure: Mix everything in a blender until you get a creamy look. Add water progressively if you want a more liquid mixture. Serve and enjoy.

Nutritional facts: Energy 256 kcal, total fat 5 g, cholesterol 8 mg, carbohydrates 72 g and fiber 7 g.

45.   Strawberry and chia juice (2 people)

Ingredients:

- 1 spoon of chia seeds
- 1 banana
- 1 ½ cup of strawberries cut in cubes
- 1 cup of milk
- 1/2 cup of ice cubes

Procedure: Mix everything in a blender until you get a creamy look. Add water progressively if you want a more liquid mixture. Serve and enjoy.

Nutritional facts: Energy 246 kcal, total fat 3 g, cholesterol 8 mg, carbohydrates 76 g and fiber 8 g.

MEALS

1.   Beet Hummus

Ingredients:

1 cup of beets, trimmed and sliced into thin slices

2 cups of chickpeas, pre-cooked

2 garlic cloves, crushed

1 tbsp of tahini

4 tbsp of olive oil

3 tbsp of lemon juice, freshly squeezed

½ tsp of salt

¼ tsp of black pepper, ground

Preparation:

Wash the beets and trim off the green ends. Cut into thin slices and set aside.

Soak the chickpeas overnight, or at least 4 hours. Cook the chickpeas until fork-tender. Remove from the heat and drain well. Set aside.

Preheat 1 tablespoon of olive oil in a large saucepan over a medium-high temperature. Add garlic and stir-fry for 2 minutes and then add beets. Cook for about 4-5 minutes, or until beets tender. Remove from the heat and set aside.

Now, combine chickpeas, beets, tahini, and lemon juice. Sprinkle with salt and pepper and gradually add olive oil while blending. Blend until smooth and creamy. If the hummus is too thick, add a bit of water to adjust it.

Serve with fresh carrots, cucumber, or celery.

Enjoy!

Nutrition information per serving: Kcal: 354, Protein: 13.9g, Carbs: 44.3g, Fats: 14.8g

2.   Trout Fillets with Tomato Sauce and Spinach

Ingredients:

1 lb trout fillets

7 oz of fresh spinach, torn

2 large tomatoes, peeled and finely chopped

4 cups of fish stock

1 tsp dried thyme, ground

½ tsp fresh rosemary, finely chopped

¼ cup olive oil

¼ cup of lime juice, freshly squeezed

1 tsp sea salt

3 garlic cloves, crushed

Preparation:

Rinse the fillets and sprinkle with sea salt.

In a large bowl, combine olive oil with thyme, rosemary, and lime juice. Stir well and submerge fillets in this mixture. Refrigerate for 30 minutes.

Remove from the refrigerator and drain the fillets but reserve the marinade.

Now use some of the marinade to grease the stainless steel cooking insert of your pressure cooker. About three tablespoons will be enough. Add fillets, fish stock, and close the lid. Set the steam release handle and press the "Fish" button. Cook for 8 minutes.

When you hear the cooker's end signal, perform a quick release and open the lid. Remove the fish and set aside.

Now add the remaining marinade into the cooker. Press the "Sautee" button and add finely chopped tomatoes. Cook until tomatoes soften. Give it a good stir and remove from the cooker.

Grease the bottom of your steel pot with some more olive oil and add garlic and spinach. Cook for five more minutes, then press "Cancel" button. Remove from the cooker and transfer to a plate. Add fish, drizzle with tomato sauce and serve warm.

Nutrition information per serving: Kcal: 479, Protein: 43.5g, Carbs: 10g, Fats: 30.2g

3.   Turkish Mixed Kebab

Ingredients:

7 oz of lean ground beef

7 oz of ground veal, tender cuts

2 large onions, peeled and finely chopped

2 garlic cloves, crushed

3 tbsp of all-purpose flour

2 tbsp of vegetable oil

1 tbsp of tomato paste

1 tbsp of fresh parsley, finely chopped

½ tsp of salt

¼ tsp of black pepper, freshly ground

2 tbsp of butter

Preparation:

In a large bowl, combine ground beef, ground veal, onions, garlic, flour, tomato paste, parsley, salt, pepper, and 1 tablespoon of oil. Mix well and shape kebabs with your hands. Set aside.

Grease the bottom of a large heavy-bottomed pot with the remaining oil. Gently place kebabs on the bottom. Add one cup of water or a beef broth. Cover with a lid and cook for 2 hours on low temperature.

Remove the kebabs from the pot and set aside.

Now, melt the butter in a large saucepan over a medium-high temperature. Add kebabs and cook for about 4-5 minutes, or until browned on each side. Serve with fresh onions and pide bread.

Nutrition information per serving: Kcal: 346, Protein: 28.9g, Carbs: 12.9g, Fats: 19.6g

4.   Kiwi Lemon Smoothie

Ingredients:

3 large kiwis, peeled

1 large lemon, juiced

1 cup of Greek yogurt

2 tbsp of fresh mint

¼ tsp of ginger, ground

1 tbsp of sunflower seeds

1 tbsp of honey, raw

1 tbsp of almonds, roughly chopped

Preparation:

Peel the kiwis. Cut lengthwise in half and transfer to a food processor. Add yogurt, mint, and ginger. Blend until nicely smooth and creamy. Transfer to serving glasses and stir in the honey and lemon juice.

Top with sunflower seeds and roughly chopped almonds.

Garnish with some fresh mint leaves and refrigerate for 20 minutes before serving.

Enjoy!

Nutrition information per serving: Kcal: 214, Protein: 12.9g, Carbs: 33.7g, Fats: 5g

5.   Sweet Pumpkin Pudding

Ingredients:

1 lb of pumpkin, peeled and chopped into bite-sized pieces

2 tbsp of honey

½ cup cornstarch

4 cups pumpkin juice, unsweetened

1 tsp cinnamon, ground

3 cloves, freshly ground

Preparation:

Peel and prepare the pumpkin. Scrape out seeds and chop into bite-sized pieces. Set aside.

In a small bowl, combine pumpkin juice, honey, orange juice, cinnamon, and cornstarch.

Place the pumpkin chops in a large pot and pour the pumpkin juice mixture. Stir well and then finally add cloves. Stir until well incorporated and heat up until almost boils. Reduce the heat to low and cook for about 15 minutes, or until the mixture thickens.

Remove from the heat and transfer to the bowls immediately. Set aside to cool completely and then refrigerate for 15 minutes before serving, or simply chill overnight.

Nutrition information per serving: Kcal: 288, Protein: 1.3g, Carbs: 74.2g, Fats: 0.3g

6.   Mango Oatmeal

Ingredients:

1 cup of rolled oats

1 cup of mango, chopped into chunks

1 cup of skim milk

1 tbsp of almonds, roughly chopped

1 tbsp of honey

¼ tsp of cinnamon, ground

1 tbsp of sunflower seeds

Preparation:

Wash and peel the mango. Cut into small chunks and set aside.

In a deep pot, combine oats, milk, and cinnamon. Heat up to over a medium-high temperature. stir in the honey and remove from the heat. Set aside and allow it to cool completely.

Now, combine oats and mango. Stir until well incorporated and top with almonds and sunflower seeds for some extra nutrients.

Enjoy!

Nutrition information per serving: Kcal: 359, Protein: 11.8g, Carbs: 68.5g, Fats: 5.6g

7.   Chicken with Garlic Lemon Sauce

Ingredients:

1 lb of chicken fillets

5 garlic cloves, minced

2 tbsp of lemon juice, freshly squeezed

1 tsp of dried oregano, ground

1 tbsp of fresh thyme, finely chopped

½ cup of white wine

3 tbsp of olive oil

½ tsp of cayenne pepper, ground

1 tsp of sea salt

¼ tsp of black pepper, ground

Preparation:

Preheat the oven to 375°F.

Wash the fillets under cold running water and pat dry with a kitchen paper. Set aside.

Preheat the oil in a small frying pan over a medium-high temperature. Add garlic and stir-fry for 2 minutes. Remove from the heat and stir in the wine, salt, pepper, cayenne, and thyme. Stir until well incorporated and pour this mixture into a large baking sheet.

Spread the chicken fillets over the sauce. Sprinkle with some additional salt and pepper and drizzle with lemon juice. Slice a few lemon slices and place them on top of the each fillet.

Bake for about 40-45 minutes, or until lightly browned.

When serving, spoon the baking sheet juices over the fillets. Serve with some fresh salad.

Nutrition information per serving: Kcal: 455, Protein: 44.4g, Carbs: 4.1g, Fats: 25.5g

8. Beet Spinach Salad

Ingredients:

2 medium-sized beet, trimmed and sliced

1 cup of fresh spinach, chopped

2 spring onions, finely chopped

1 small green apple, cored and chopped

3 tbsp of olive oil

2 tbsp of fresh lime juice

1 tbsp of honey, raw

1 tsp of apple cider vinegar

1 tsp of salt

Preparation:

Wash the beets and trim off the green parts. Set aside.

Wash the spinach thoroughly and drain. Cut into small pieces and set aside.

Wash the apple and cut lengthwise in half. Remove the core and cut into bite-sized pieces and set aside.

Wash the onions and cut into small pieces. Set aside.

In a small bowl, combine olive oil, lime juice, honey, vinegar, and salt. Stir until well incorporated and set aside to allow flavors to meld.

Place the beets in a deep pot. Pour enough water to cover and cook for about 40 minutes, or until tender. Remove the skin and slice. Set aside.

In a large salad bowl, combine beets, spinach, spring onions, and apple. Stir well until combined and drizzle with previously prepared dressing. Give it a good final stir and serve immediately.

Nutrition information per serving: Kcal: 324, Protein: 2.7g, Carbs: 36.1g, Fats: 21.5g

9.   Carrot Lentil Soup

Ingredients:

1 cup of red lentils, soaked

4 large carrots, peeled and chopped

1 medium-sized onion, peeled and finely chopped

3 tbsp of milk

1 tbsp of all-purpose flour

½ tsp of black pepper, freshly ground

½ tsp of cumin, ground

½ tsp of salt

2 tbsp of olive oil

Preparation:

Wash and peel the carrots. Place them in a food processor and add milk. Blend until smooth and creamy. Set aside.

Soak the lentils overnight. Rinse well and drain. Place in a deep pot of boiling water and cook for 15 minutes. Remove from the heat and drain. Set aside.

Preheat the oil in a large saucepan over a medium-high temperature. Add onions and flour. Stir-fry for 5 minutes, or until translucent.

Now, add carrot puree and lentils. Sprinkle with salt and pepper to taste and stir well. Cook for 1 minute and then add 4 cups of water. Stir well and bring it to a boil. Reduce the heat to low and cook for 1 hour. Remove from the heat and serve warm.

Sprinkle with some fresh parsley before serving. However, this is optional.

Nutrition information per serving: Kcal: 284, Protein: 13.9g, Carbs: 40.8g, Fats: 7.9g

10.   Creamy Basil Portobello Mushrooms

Ingredients:

3 large Portobello mushrooms

4 cups of fresh basil, chopped

½ tsp of dried rosemary, ground

½ cup of Greek yogurt

1 tbsp of balsamic vinegar

4 tbsp of olive oil

¼ tsp black pepper, ground

½ tsp of sea salt

Preparation:

Preheat the oven to 450°F.

In a medium bowl, combine oil, vinegar, rosemary, and salt. Stir until well incorporated and set aside.

Wash the mushrooms and remove the stems. Cut into bite-sized pieces and place in a large saucepan. Pour over the previously prepared sauce and stir until combined. Soak the mushrooms for 20 minutes and then transfer to a large baking dish. Reserve the sauce for later.

Place it in the oven and bake for about 13-15 minutes. Remove from the heat and transfer to a serving plate.

Combine basil and yogurt and stir well. Sprinkle with some salt if you like and serve with mushrooms.

Drizzle all with reserved sauce and serve immediately.

Nutrition information per serving: Kcal: 322, Protein: 11.1g, Carbs: 8.2g, Fats: 29.4g

11. Carrot Onion Omelet

Ingredients:

3 large eggs, beaten

3 spring onions, finely chopped

3 baby carrots, thinly sliced

¼ tsp of salt

¼ tsp of cayenne pepper

2 tbsp of extra-virgin olive oil

Preparation:

Heat up the olive oil in a frying skillet over a medium-high temperature. Add onions and carrots. Fry for about 3-4 minutes, stirring occasionally.

Meanwhile, beat the eggs in a medium bowl. Sprinkle with some salt and pepper to taste.

Pour the egg mixture over the vegetables and cook for about 3-4 minutes. using a large wooden spoon or spatula, flip the omelet. Cook for 1 more minute and remove from the heat.

Serve immediately.

Nutrition information per serving: Kcal: 240, Protein: 10g, Carbs: 3.6g, Fats: 21.6g

12.   Garlic Chicken Breast

Ingredients:

2 lbs chicken breast, skinless and boneless

1 ½ cups chicken broth

4 garlic cloves, crushed

2 tbsp of olive oil

1 medium-sized onion, peeled and finely chopped

½ tbsp of garlic powder

1 tsp of salt

¼ tsp of black pepper, ground

Preparation:

Wash the chicken breasts under cold running water and pat dry with a kitchen paper. Set aside.

Preheat the oil in a large skillet over a medium-high temperature. Add onions and stir-fry for about 3-4 minutes, or until translucent. Add garlic and cook for 1 more minute.

Now, add all other ingredients and bring it to a boil. Reduce the heat to low and cover with a lid. Taste and add more salt if needed. Cook for about 20-25 minutes, or until set.

Remove from the heat and sprinkle with some fresh parsley before serving. Serve with steamed vegetables or rice. However, this is optional.

Nutrition information per serving: Kcal: 236, Protein: 20g, Carbs: 6.3g, Fats: 14.5g

13.   Grilled Avocado in Curry Sauce

Ingredients:

1 large avocado, chopped

¼ cup of water

1 tbsp of curry, ground

2 tbsp of olive oil

1 tsp of soy sauce

1 tsp of fresh parsley, finely chopped

¼ tsp of red pepper flakes

¼ tsp of sea salt

Preparation:

Peel the avocado and cut lengthwise in half. Remove the pit and cut into small chunks. Set aside.

Heat up the olive oil in a large saucepan over a medium-high temperature.

In a small bowl, combine ground curry, soy sauce, parsley, red pepper and sea salt. Add water and cook for about 5 minutes, stirring occasionally.

Add chopped avocado, stir well and cook for 3 more minutes, or until all the liquid evaporates. Turn off the heat and cover. Let it stand for about 15-20 minutes before serving.

Nutrition information per serving: Kcal: 338, Protein: 2.5g, Carbs: 10.8g, Fats: 34.1g

14.   Green and Kidney Beans Salad

Ingredients:

1 cup of cooked green beans

½ cup of kidney beans

¼ cup of sweet corn

1 small onion, peeled

1 cup of lettuce, chopped

1 green bell pepper, chopped

5 tbsp of orange juice

1 tbsp of olive oil

½ tsp of salt

Preparation:

Wash the green beans and cut into bite-sized pieces. Place them in a pot of boiling water and cook for 15 minutes. Remove from the heat and drain well. Set aside.

Soak the kidney beans overnight. Rinse well and drain. Place them in a pot of boiling water and cook for 20 minutes. Remove from the heat and drain well. Set aside.

Wash the green pepper and cut lengthwise in half. Remove the seeds and chop into small pieces. Set aside.

Wash the lettuce thoroughly under cold running water and roughly chop it. Place it in a large salad bowl. Add peeled and finely chopped onions, green beans, kidney beans, corn, and pepper.

In a small bowl, combine orange juice, oil, and salt. Stir well and drizzle over the salad. Toss well to coat all the ingredients and serve immediately.

You can add some orange wedges if you like, but this is optional.

Enjoy!

Nutrition information per serving: Kcal: 303, Protein: 13.4g, Carbs: 48.4g, Fats: 8.1g

15.   Pumpkin Porridge

Ingredients:

1 cup of pumpkin, chopped

1 cup of fresh arugula, chopped

3 tbsp of almonds, chopped

1 tsp of dry rosemary, finely chopped

½ tsp of dry thyme, ground

1 tbsp of olive oil

Preparation:

Preheat the oven to 350°F.

Peel the pumpkin and cut lengthwise in half. Scrape out the seeds and one large wedge. Cut into chunks and fill the measuring cup. Wrap the rest of the pumpkin in a plastic foil and refrigerate for later.

Grease a large baking sheet with the olive oil. Spread the pumpkin and sprinkle with rosemary and thyme. Bake for about 30 minutes. Remove from the oven and allow it to cool for a while.

Meanwhile, combine all other ingredients in a bowl. Add baked pumpkin and drizzle with some more olive oil. Stir all well and serve.

Nutrition information per serving: Kcal: 317, Protein: 7.1g, Carbs: 25.5g, Fats: 24g

16.   Hazelnut Quinoa

Ingredients:

1 cup of quinoa, cooked

3 tbsp of hazelnuts, roasted

1 cup of button mushrooms, sliced

¼ cup of prunes, chopped

½ cup of fresh parsley, finely chopped

1 small onion, peeled and chopped

2 garlic cloves, crushed

¼ tsp of salt

4 tbsp of olive oil

Preparation:

Combine 3 tablespoons of olive oil, parsley, and hazelnuts in a food processor. Blend well for 30 seconds and set aside.

Heat up the remaining olive oil in a large skillet. Add chopped onion and garlic. Stir well and fry for several minutes, until nice golden color.

Add cooked quinoa, button mushrooms, and mix well. Cook for 5 more minutes, until the water evaporates.

Remove from the heat and transfer to a bowl. Add hazelnut mixture and ¼ cup of cranberries.

Mix well and serve warm.

Nutrition information per serving: Kcal: 453, Protein: 10.4g, Carbs: 50.4g, Fats: 25.2g

17.　Chili Smoothie

Ingredients:

2 large red bell peppers, chopped

1 medium-sized tomato, chopped

1 cup of fresh broccoli, chopped

1 cup of Greek yogurt

½ tsp of dried oregano, ground

½ tsp of salt

¼ tsp of chili pepper, ground

1 tbsp of fresh lemon juice

Preparation:

Wash the bell peppers and cut lengthwise in half. Remove the seeds and chop into small pieces. Set aside.

Wash the tomato and gently peel it. Cut into bite-sized pieces. Make sure to reserve the juice while cutting. Set aside.

Wash the broccoli and cut into small pieces. Set aside.

Now, combine bell peppers, tomato, broccoli, yogurt, oregano, salt, and lemon juice in a food processor. Blend until nicely smooth and transfer to serving glasses.

Refrigerate for 15 minutes before serving.

Nutrition information per serving: Kcal: 143, Protein: 13.2g, Carbs: 18.9g, Fats: 2.7g

18. Lemon Rolls

Ingredients:

1 cup of basmati rice

2 cherry tomatoes, finely chopped

¼ cup of red bell pepper, finely chopped

1 tbsp of tomato paste

2 tbsp of lime juice, freshly squeezed

1 bunch of collard greens, whole leaves

1 tbsp of olive oil

½ tsp of salt

¼ tsp of black pepper, ground

Preparation:

Wash the collard greens under cold running water and drain. Briefly, boil the collard greens for 2 minutes. Remove from the heat and drain. Set aside.

Wash the tomatoes and bell pepper. Dice the tomatoes and set aside. Cut the bell pepper lengthwise in half and remove the seeds. Cut into small pieces and set aside.

Now, combine rice, diced tomatoes, bell peppers, tomato paste, and lime juice. Sprinkle with some salt and pepper and stir until well incorporated.

Spread the collard greens on a clean surface and use one tablespoon of mixture for each roll. Roll and tuck in the ends while rolling.

Now, preheat the oil in a deep pot over a medium-high temperature. Place the rolls and add about ½ cup of water. Cover with a lid and cook for about 30 minutes.

Nutrition information per serving: Kcal: 447, Protein: 9.3g, Carbs: 84.9g, Fats: 8.3g

19. Spinach Veal Soup

Ingredients:

1 lb of veal steak, cut into bite-sized pieces

1 lb of fresh spinach, torn

3 large eggs, beaten

4 cups of vegetable broth

1 small onion, finely chopped

2 garlic cloves

3 tbsp of extra-virgin olive oil

1 tsp of salt

Preparation:

Wash the meat under cold running water and pat dry with a kitchen paper. Cut into bite-sized pieces and place in a medium bowl. Generously sprinkle with salt and pepper and stir well with your hands. Set aside.

Rinse spinach thoroughly and drain. Cut into bite-sized pieces and set aside.

Preheat the oil in a large skillet over a medium-high temperature. Add meat and cook for 5 minutes, stirring occasionally. Add garlic and onions and give it a good stir. Cook for another 3-4 minutes, or until the onions translucent.

Now, add vegetable broth and spinach. Bring it to a boil and then whisk in the eggs. Reduce the heat to low and cook for about an hour. Remove from the heat and serve immediately.

Nutrition information per serving: Kcal: 333, Protein: 34.4g, Carbs: 6g, Fats: 19.1g

20.   Frozen Raspberry Cream

Ingredients:

1 cup of almond cream

1 cup of fresh raspberry

¼ cup of skim milk

1 tbsp of cherry extract

2 tbsp of honey, raw

Preparation:

Wash the raspberries using a large colander. Drain and set aside.

Combine the ingredients in a large bowl. Beat with a fork until well incorporated. Use popsicles, plastic glasses, or paper cups and make an ice cream. However, this is optional.

Put it in a freezer for about 30 minutes. Garnish with some nuts or add a teaspoon of lemon juice for some extra nutrients and flavor.

Enjoy!

Nutrition information per serving: Kcal: 265, Protein: 9.4g, Carbs: 61.4g, Fats: 0.1g

21.   Broccoli Cauliflower Puree

Ingredients:

2 cups of fresh broccoli chopped

2 cups of fresh cauliflower, chopped

½ cup of skim milk

½ tsp of salt

½ tsp of Italian seasoning

¼ tsp of cumin, ground

1 tbsp of fresh parsley, finely chopped

1 tbsp of olive oil

1 tsp of dry mint, ground

Preparation:

Wash and roughly chop the cauliflower. Place it in a deep pot and add a pinch of salt. Cook for about 15-20 minutes. When done, drain and transfer it to a food processor. Set aside.

Wash the broccoli and chop into bite-sized pieces. Add it to the food processor along with milk, salt, Italian seasoning, cumin, parsley, and mint. Gradually add olive oil and blend until nicely pureed.

Serve with some fresh carrots and celery.

Nutrition information per serving: Kcal: 266, Protein: 12.3g, Carbs: 25.5g, Fats: 15.1g

22. Vegetable Dziugas Salad

Ingredients:

1 cup of cherry tomatoes

½ cup of dziugas cheese, sliced

½ cup of lamb's spinach

1 small orange

1 tbsp of Parmesan cheese

1 tsp of fresh lemon juice

Preparation:

Wash the tomatoes and cut in half. Set aside.

Wash the spinach thoroughly under cold running water and chop into small pieces. Set aside.

Peel the orange and divide into wedges. Cut each wedge in half and set aside.

Now, combine tomatoes, spinach, and orange. Top with cheese and drizzle with lemon juice before serving. Enjoy!

Nutrition information per serving: Kcal: 210, Protein: 13.7g, Carbs: 11.3g, Fats: 12.9g

23. Poached Eggs with Spinach

Ingredients:

4 large eggs, beaten

1 cup of fresh spinach, chopped

½ cup of Greek yogurt

2 garlic cloves, finely chopped

1 small onion, finely chopped

1 tbsp of olive oil

1 tsp of salt

¼ tsp of black pepper, ground

Preparation:

Wash the spinach thoroughly under cold running water. Drain and chop into bite-sized pieces.

Peel the onion and garlic. Finely chop it and set aside.

Place the spinach in a deep pot. Add 2 cups of water and sprinkle with some salt. Bring it to a boil and cook for 3 more minutes. Remove from the heat and drain well. Set aside.

Now, preheat the oil in a large frying pan over a medium-high temperature. Add onions and garlic. Stir-fry for 2 minutes, or until translucent. Crack the eggs and add it directly to the pan. Do not stir. Cook for about 4-5 minutes, or until the egg whites thicken. Sprinkle with some salt and pepper to taste and remove from the heat.

Serve with yogurt and enjoy!

Nutrition information per serving: Kcal: 263, Protein: 18.7g, Carbs: 7.8g, Fats: 18.1g

24.   Vegan Wok Veggies

Ingredients:

1 medium red pepper, cut into strips

1 medium green pepper, cut into strips

7-8 pieces of baby corn

½ cup of button mushrooms, canned

1 cup of cauliflower, chopped into bite-sized pieces

1 medium carrot, peeled and cut into strips

1 tsp of oyster sauce

1 tbsp of olive oil

1 tsp of sea salt

Preparation:

Wash and prepare the vegetables. Set aside.

In a large wok, heat up the olive oil over a medium-high temperature. Add carrots and cauliflower.Keep in mind that some vegetables take more time to cook.Cook for about 8-10 minutes.

Now, add red and green pepper strips, baby corn, button mushrooms, and oyster sauce. Cook for another 5-7 minutes. You don't want to overcook the vegetables. Vegetables in wok should be nice and crispy.

You can serve your vegetables with rice, pasta, or boiled potatoes. I like to serve it with standard white rice sprinkled with turmeric. Brown rice pasta is also a very nice side dish for this lunch.

Nutrition information per serving: Kcal: 388, Protein: 13.6g, Carbs: 76.7g, Fats: 9.1g

25.   Blueberry Parfait

Ingredients:

2 cups of skim milk

2 tbsp of cream, low fat

1 large egg

2 egg whites

1 tbsp of honey

½ cup of fresh blueberries

½ tsp of vanilla extract

Preparation:

Gently warm the milk over a low heat. Add the cream and stir constantly. You don't want it to boil. Remove from the heat and set aside. Allow it to cool completely.

Using a hand mixer, stir in the egg, egg whites, honey, and blueberries. Pour the parfait into tall glasses and top with some fresh blueberries.

Freeze overnight before serving.

Nutrition information per serving: Kcal: 206, Protein: 15.2g, Carbs: 26.8g, Fats: 3.4g

26. Bean Tomato Soup

Ingredients:

2 lbs of medium-sized tomatoes, pureed

1 cup of kidney beans, pre-cooked

1 small onion, diced

2 garlic cloves, crushed

1 cup of heavy cream

1 cup of vegetable broth

2 tbsp of fresh parsley, finely chopped

¼ tsp of black pepper, ground

2 tbsp of extra-virgin olive oil

1 tsp of dry oregano, ground

½ tsp of salt

¼ tsp of chili pepper, ground

Preparation:

Soak the beans overnight. Rinse and drain well and place the beans in a deep pot. Add 4 cups of water and bring it to a boil. Cook for 30 minutes and then remove from the heat. Drain and set aside.

Wash the tomatoes and cut into bite-sized pieces. Transfer to a food processor and add some salt and oregano. Blend until smooth and creamy and set aside.

Now, preheat the oil in a large saucepan over a medium-high temperature. Add onions and garlic and stir-fry for 5 minutes, or until translucent. Add beans, tomatoes, and broth. Stir well and bring it to a boil. Reduce the heat to low and sprinkle with chili. Stir well and cook for 35-40 minutes. Add heavy cream and cook for 2 more minutes, stirring constantly.

Remove from the heat and sprinkle with parsley before serving.

Nutrition information per serving: Kcal: 358, Protein: 13g, Carbs: 42.8g, Fats: 15.2g

27.   White Beans Pepper Salad

Ingredients:

1 cup of white beans, pre-cooked

1 red bell pepper, chopped into bite-sized pieces

1 tsp of fresh parsley, finely chopped

1 tbsp of olive oil

1 tbsp of lemon juice, freshly squeezed

½ tsp of dried mint, ground

½ tsp of sea salt

Preparation:

Soak the beans overnight. Rinse well with cold water and drain. Place in a deep pot and add 3 cups of water. Bring it to a boil and then cook for 20 minutes. Remove from the heat and drain. Set aside.

Wash the bell pepper and cut lengthwise in half. Remove the seeds and chop into bite-sized pieces. Set aside.

In a large salad bowl, combine cooked beans, bell pepper, and fresh parsley, Drizzle with olive oil and lemon juice.

Sprinkle with salt and mint to taste before serving.

Nutrition information per serving: Kcal: 418, Protein: 24.3g, Carbs: 65.6g, Fats: 8.1g

28.   Spinach Lime Smoothie

Ingredients:

2 cups of fresh spinach, chopped

1 medium-sized lime, peeled

¼ tsp of ginger, ground

2 tbsp of almonds

1 cup of skim milk

Preparation:

Wash the spinach thoroughly under cold running water. Drain and chop into small pieces. Place the spinach in a pot of boiling water. Sprinkle with salt and cook for 2 minutes. Remove from the heat and drain well. Set aside.

Peel the lime and cut lengthwise in half. Set aside.

Now, combine spinach, lime, ginger and milk in a food processor or a blender. Process until smooth and creamy. Transfer to serving glasses and top with almonds.

Add some ice cubes and serve immediately.

Nutrition information per serving: Kcal: 97, Protein: 6.4g, Carbs: 12.1g, Fats: 3.2g

29. Grilled Lemon Shrimps

Ingredients:

1 lb of fresh shrimps, cleaned

1 tbsp of fresh rosemary, for serving

4 tbsp extra-virgin olive oil

1 tsp of garlic powder

2 tbsp of lemon juice, freshly squeezed

½ tsp of salt

½ tsp of black pepper, freshly ground

½ tsp of dried thyme, ground

½ tsp of dried oregano, ground

1 organic lemon, sliced into wedges, for serving

Preparation:

Combine olive oil, garlic, lemon juice, salt, pepper, thyme, and oregano in a medium bowl and mix until well incorporated. Place the shrimp and coat evenly with the marinade mixture. Cover the bowl and chill for at least 1 hour to marinate the shrimps.

Preheat the grill to a medium-high temperature. Brush the grill grids with some oil.

Insert 2 to 3 shrimps on each skewer, brush with marinade and grill for 3 minutes. Turn and grill the other side for another 3 minutes. Transfer to a serving platter.

Serve warm with lemons wedges and sprinkle with chopped parsley.

Nutrition information per serving: Kcal: 532, Protein: 52.4g, Carbs: 8.7g, Fats: 32.4g

30.　Mushroom Rice Salad

Ingredients:

½ cup of rice, long-grained

1 cup of fresh button mushrooms, chopped

½ cup of fresh broccoli, chopped

1 tbsp of olive oil

2 tbsp of vegetable oil

1 tbsp of dried rosemary, finely chopped

1 tsp of lime juice, freshly squeezed

½ tsp of salt

¼ tsp of black pepper, freshly ground

Preparation:

Wash and rinse the rice and put in a saucepan with 1 cup of water. Stir well and bring to the boiling point. Cover the pan with a lid and cook for about 15 minutes over a low temperature. Remove from the heat and allow it to cool.

Wash and cut the mushrooms into bite-size pieces.

Heat up the oil in a large saucepan over a medium-high temperature. Add mushrooms and stir well. Cook for 2 minutes and then add broccoli. Cook for 5 minutes more until soften, or until all the water evaporates. Remove from the frying pan. Add salt and mix with rice and broccoli.

Season with rosemary, pepper and lime juice. Serve warm.

Nutrition information per serving: Kcal: 372, Protein: 5.2g, Carbs: 41.3g, Fats: 21.4g

31. Cheesy Turkey

Ingredients:

1 lb of turkey breasts, boneless and skinless

½ cup of cheddar cheese, grated

1 cup of fresh arugula, chopped

1 large tomato, finely chopped

½ cup of button mushrooms, sliced

1 small zucchini, chopped

1 tsp of salt

¼ tsp of red pepper, ground

2 tbsp of olive oil

Preparation:

Wash and pat dry the meat with some kitchen paper. Cut into bite-sized pieces and set aside.

Wash the arugula under cold running water and roughly chop it. Set aside.

Peel and chop the zucchini into small pieces. Set aside.

Preheat the oil in a large grill pan over a medium-high temperature. Add turkey chops and cook for 5 minutes, or until lightly browned. Add mushrooms and zucchini and sprinkle with some salt and pepper to taste. Cook for another 7 minutes, stirring occasionally. Remove from the heat and set aside.

In a large salad bowl, combine tomato and arugula. Stir to combine and add turkey mix. Taste and add more salt and pepper if needed. Top with cheese and serve.

I like to drizzle with some lemon juice, but this is optional.

Enjoy!

Nutrition information per serving: Kcal: 338, Protein: 32.2g, Carbs: 11.7g, Fats: 18.4g

32.　　Marinated Tuna

Ingredients:

2 lbs of tuna steaks, boneless

¼ cup of fresh coriander, chopped

2 garlic cloves, minced

2 tablespoons of lemon juice

1 cup olive oil

½ tsp of smoked paprika

½ tsp of cumin, ground

½ tsp of chili pepper, ground

½ tsp of salt

¼ tsp of black pepper, ground

Preparation:

Add the coriander, garlic, paprika, cumin, chili and lemon juice in a food processor and pulse to combine. Gradually add in the oil and mix the ingredients until a smooth mixture.

Transfer the mixture into a bowl, add the fish and gently toss to coat the fish evenly with sauce. Chill for at least 2 hours to allow the flavors to penetrate into the fish.

Remove the fish from the chiller and preheat the grill. Lightly brush the grid with oil, place the fish and grill for about 3 to 4 minutes on each side.

Remove the fish from the grill, transfer to a serving plate and serve with lemon wedges or some vegetables.

Nutrition information per serving: Kcal: 514, Protein: 68.1g, Carbs: 1.1g, Fats: 24.9g

33.   Kiwi Banana Oatmeal

Ingredients:

2 large kiwis, peeled

1 large banana

1 cup of rolled oats

1 cup of milk

1 tbsp of chia seeds

1/4 cup of raisins

1 tbsp of honey, raw

1 tbsp of almonds, roughly chopped

Preparation:

Peel the kiwis and banana. Cut into thin slices and set aside.

Heat up the milk in a deep pot to a medium-high temperature, but do not boil. Remove from the heat and stir in the rolled oats. Stir until well incorporated and set aside to soak for 15 minutes.

Now, stir in the raisins, honey, and chia seeds. Top with kiwi and banana and sprinkle with almonds.

Serve immediately.

Nutrition information per serving: Kcal: 487, Protein: 14.7g, Carbs: 88.6g, Fats: 10.7g

34.   Veal Stew

Ingredients:

2 lbs of veal, cut into bite-sized pieces

¾ cup of red wine

1 tbsp of vegetable oil

6 oz of tomato paste

2 medium-sized carrots, cut into strips

1 large tomato, chopped

1 large onion, chopped

1 cup of button mushrooms

¼ tbsp of salt

2 ½ cups beef broth

1 tsp of dry thyme

3 minced garlic cloves

1 bay leaf

Preparation:

Wash the meat under cold running water and pat dry with

a kitchen paper. Cut into bite-sized pieces and set aside.

Preheat the oil in a large frying pan over a medium-high temperature. Add meat chops and cook for 8-10 minutes, or until browned. Now, remove from the heat and transfer meat to a heavy-bottomed pot. Reserve the pan.

Add onions to the pan and stir-fry for about 3-4 minutes, or until translucent. Add wine and tomato paste and stir until well incorporated. Cook for 3 minutes more and remove from the heat. Pour this mixture into the pot with meat. Add the remaining ingredients and cover with a lid. Bring it all to boil and then reduce the heat to low. Cook for about an hour.

Remove from the heat and serve warm.

Nutrition information per serving: Kcal: 373, Protein: 41.3g, Carbs: 13.1g, Fats: 14.5g

35. Salmon with Yogurt Marinade

Ingredients:

1 lb of fresh salmon, cut into bite-sized pieces

1 cup of sour cream

1 cup of Greek yogurt

3 garlic cloves, crushed

2 large eggs

½ tsp of sea salt

1 tbsp of dry parsley

2 tbsp of extra-virgin olive oil

Preparation:

Preheat the oven to 350°F.

Combine the sour cream, Greek yogurt, eggs, garlic, salt, and dry parsley in a bowl. Place salmon slices in this marinade and cover with a lid. Marinate for about an hour.

Now transfer the salmon slices in a small baking dish. Place it in the oven and bake for 30 minutes.

Remove from the oven and drizzle with the remaining marinade.

Serve the salmon with steamed asparagus, or boiled potato and spinach, however, this is optional.

Enjoy!

Nutrition information per serving: Kcal: 410, Protein: 32.2g, Carbs: 5.5g, Fats: 29.6g

36. Chicken Rice Casserole

Ingredients:

1 lb of chicken thighs

1 cup of brown rice

3 cups of chicken broth

1 small onion, chopped

1 large carrot, chopped

½ cup of artichoke, cooked

½ cup of green beans, cooked and drained

½ tsp of salt

¼ tsp of black pepper, ground

Preparation:

Preheat oven to 250°F.

Combine the chicken and onions into a skillet and cook over a medium-high heat until chicken is cooked. This should take about 20-30 minutes. Remove from the heat and drain, but keep the liquid. Set the meat aside.

Place the onions into a large bowl and then add brown rice, vegetables, salt, and pepper. Add the chicken broth. Mix up until everything is thoroughly combined.

Place the mixture into an ungreased 1½ quart casserole dish with a tight-fitting lid.

Bake covered for about 30 minutes, or until rice is done, stirring it several times during cooking.

Uncover the casserole dish and add chicken thighs.

Bake uncovered for about 5 more minutes until nicely golden brown color.

Nutrition information per serving: Kcal: 387, Protein: 27.3g, Carbs: 43g, Fats: 12.4g

37.   Broccoli Gorgonzola Soup

Ingredients:

10 oz of Gorgonzola cheese, crumbled

1 cup of broccoli, finely chopped

1 tbsp of olive oil

½ cup of full-fat milk

½ cup of vegetable broth

1 tbsp of parsley, finely chopped

½ tsp of salt

¼ tsp of black pepper, ground

Preparation:

Wash the broccoli under cold running water. Drain and chop into bite-sized pieces. Set aside.

Grease the bottom of a deep pot with olive oil. Add all ingredients and three cups of water. Mix well with a kitchen whisker until fully combined.

Cover with a lid and cook for 2 hours on low temperature.

Remove from the heat and sprinkle with some fresh parsley for extra taste.

I like to stir in one tablespoon of Greek yogurt before serving, but it's optional.

Nutrition information per serving: Kcal: 208, Protein: 11.8g, Carbs: 7.6g, Fats: 15.8g

38. Vegetarian Paella

Ingredients:

½ cup of fresh green peas

2 small carrots, finely chopped

1 cup of fire-roasted tomatoes

1 cup of zucchini, finely chopped

½ cup of celery root, finely chopped

8 saffron threads

1 tbsp of turmeric, ground

1 tsp of salt

½ tsp of freshly ground black pepper

2 cup of vegetable broth

1 cup of long grain rice

Preparation:

Combine all ingredients, except rice, in a deep pot. Stir well and cover with a lid. Bring it to a boil and then reduce the heat to low. Cook for 3 hours, or until peas are tender.

Stir in rice and again cover with the lid. Cook for 15-20 more minutes. Remove from the heat.

Optionally, sprinkle with some fresh parsley. Serve warm.

Nutrition information per serving: Kcal: 235, Protein: 7.9g, Carbs: 47g, Fats: 1.4g

39.   Sweet Potato Kefir Smoothie

Ingredients:

1 medium-sized sweet potato, chopped

2 medium-sized carrots, chopped

1 cup of kefir, low-fat

½ tsp of ginger, ground

¼ tsp of salt

2 tbsp of orange juice, freshly squeezed

Preparation:

Peel the sweet potato and cut into chunks. Place it in a pot of boiling water and sprinkle with some salt. Cook for 10 minutes and remove from the heat. Drain well and set aside.

Peel and wash the carrots. Cut into thin slices and set aside.

Now, combine potatoes, carrots, kefir, ginger, and orange juice in a food processor. Blend until nicely smooth and transfer to serving glasses.

Refrigerate for about 10-15 minutes. Garnish with some fresh mint before serving. However, it's optional.

Nutrition information per serving: Kcal: 172, Protein: 8.8g, Carbs: 32.2g, Fats: 1.2g

40.   Braised Swiss Chard

Ingredients:

1 lb of Swiss chard, torn (keep the stems)

2 medium-sized potatoes, peeled and finely chopped

3 tbsp of extra-virgin olive oil

1 small onion, chopped

2 garlic cloves, finely chopped

1 tsp of salt

¼ tsp of black pepper, ground

Preparation:

Wash the Swiss chard thoroughly under cold running water. Torn with hands and set aside.

Place Swiss chard in a large, heavy-bottomed pot. Add enough water to cover and bring it to a boil. Briefly cook, for about 3 minutes until greens are tender. Drain in a colander and set aside.

Preheat the oil in a large skillet over a medium-high temperature. Add onions and garlic and stir-fry for about 3-4 minutes, or until translucent. Add potatoes and 1 cup of water. Bring it to a boil and reduce the heat to low. Cook for 15 minutes, or until water evaporates. Add Swiss chard and sprinkle with some salt and pepper. Cook for 2 more minutes and then remove from the heat.

Serve immediately.

Nutrition information per serving: Kcal: 390, Protein: 8.3g, Carbs: 46.4g, Fats: 21.9g

41. Mixed Fish Stew

Ingredients:

2 lb of different fish and seafood

4 tbsp of extra-virgin olive oil

2 large onions, peeled and finely chopped

2 large carrots, grated

A handful of fresh parsley, finely chopped

3 garlic cloves, crushed

3 cups of water

1 tsp of sea salt

Preparation:

Preheat the oil in a large skillet over a medium-high temperature. Add onions and garlic and stir-fry for about 3-4 minutes, or until translucent.

Now, add fish mix and water. Bring it to a boil and then reduce the heat to low. Add carrots and parsley and sprinkle with some salt. Stir all well and cook for 30 minutes.

Sprinkle with a few drops of freshly squeezed lemon juice before serving, but this is optional.

Nutrition information per serving: Kcal: 504, Protein: 37.2g, Carbs: 8.1g, Fats: 35.5g

42.　Cold Cauliflower Salad

Ingredients:

1 lb of cauliflower florets

1 lb of fresh broccoli

4 garlic cloves, crushed

¼ cup of extra-virgin olive oil

1 tsp of salt

1 tbsp of dry rosemary, crushed

Preparation:

Rinse and drain the cauliflower and broccoli. Cut into bite-sized pieces and place in a deep pot. Add olive oil and one cup of water. Season with salt, crushed garlic, and dry rosemary. Bring it to a boil and then reduce the heat to low. Cover with a lid and cook for 30 minutes and then remove from the heat.

Chill well before serving.

Nutrition information per serving: Kcal: 182, Protein: 5.7g, Carbs: 15.1g, Fats: 13.2g

43.   Stuffed Avocado

Ingredients:

2 medium-sized ripe avocados, cut in half

6 large eggs

1 medium-sized tomato, finely chopped

3 tbsp of olive oil

2 tbsp of fresh parsley, finely chopped

4 tbsp of Greek Yogurt

1 tbsp of fresh rosemary, finely chopped

½ tsp of salt

¼ tsp of black pepper, ground

Preparation:

Preheat oven to 350°F. Grease a small baking dish with some oil and set aside.

Cut avocado in half and scrape out the flesh from the center. Set aside.

In a medium bowl, whisk the eggs, tomatoes, parsley, rosemary, salt, and pepper. Stir until well incorporated. Spoon this mixture into avocado shells.

Spread the stuffed avocado on the baking sheet. Make sure to avocados fit tightly. Place it in the oven and bake for about 15-20 minutes.

Remove from the heat and top with yogurt and serve.

Nutrition information per serving: Kcal: 421, Protein: 13g, Carbs: 11.7g, Fats: 38g

44. Mexican Tostadas

Ingredients:

1lb of chicken fillets, cut into bite-sized pieces

1 cup of cherry tomatoes, cut in half

1 large red bell pepper, chopped

½ cup of sweet corn, cooked

2 tbsp of fresh lemon juice

1 tsp of garlic powder

1 tsp of dry oregano, ground

3 tbsp of olive oil

¼ tsp of chili pepper, ground

½ tsp of salt

¼ tsp of black pepper, ground

4 tortillas

Preparation:

Wash the meat under cold running water and pat dry with a kitchen paper. Cut into bite-sized pieces and set aside.

Wash the bell pepper and cut lengthwise in half. Remove the seeds and cut into small pieces. Set aside.

Wash the tomatoes and cut in half. Set aside.

Now, combine peppers, tomatoes, and corn. Sprinkle with lemon juice, garlic powder, and salt. Toss well to blend and set aside.

Preheat the oil in a large skillet over a medium-high temperature. Add chicken chops and sprinkle with oregano, garlic, chili, salt, and pepper. Cook for about 10 minutes, or until nicely golden brown. Remove from the heat and set aside.

Spoon the vegetable mixture and chicken to each tortilla evenly. Wrap and secure each tortilla with a toothpick.

Serve immediately.

Nutrition information per serving: Kcal: 399, Protein: 35.8g, Carbs: 19.5g, Fats: 20.1g

45.   Quinoa Apple Porridge

Ingredients:

1 cup of quinoa

2 cups of water

1 large green apple, cut into bite-sized pieces

¼ tsp of cinnamon

1 tbsp of fresh mint, chopped

1 tbsp of nuts, roughly chopped

1 tbsp of honey

Preparation:

Wash the apple and cut lengthwise in half. Remove the core and cut into bite-sized pieces. Set aside.

Place quinoa in a deep pot. Add water and bring it to a boil. Reduce the heat to low and cook for 15 minutes. Remove from the heat and fluff with a fork. Set aside for 10 minutes.

Stir in the cinnamon and honey. Top with apple chops and sprinkle with nuts and mint.

Nutrition information per serving: Kcal: 398, Protein: 13.1g, Carbs: 71.5g, Fats: 7.6g

46.   Eggplant Tomato Stew

Ingredients:

2 medium-sized eggplants, sliced

1 medium-sized onion, peeled and chopped

2 medium-sized tomatoes, roughly chopped

1 medium-sized celery stalk, chopped

2 oz of capers

 2 tbsp of extra-virgin olive oil

1 tbsp of balsamic vinegar

½ tsp of dried basil, ground

1 tsp of salt

Preparation:

Wash the eggplants and chop into bite-sized pieces. Sprinkle with some salt and allow it to stand for about 30 minutes.

Peel the onion and finely chop it. Set aside.

Wash the tomatoes and cut into bite-sized pieces. Set aside.

Wash the celery and cut into small pieces. Set aside.

Now, preheat the oil in a large skillet over a medium-high temperature. Add onions and stir-fry for about 3-4 minutes, or until translucent. Add eggplant chops and cook for 5 more minutes, stirring occasionally. Add tomatoes, celery, vinegar, capers, and basil Stir all well and add 2 cups of water.

Bring it to a boil and then reduce the heat to low. Cover with a lid and cook for 2 hours. Remove from the heat and serve warm.

Nutrition information per serving: Kcal: 193, Protein: 4.7g, Carbs: 25.9g, Fats: 10.3g

47.   Strawberry Orange Salad

Ingredients:

1 cup of fresh strawberries, chopped

1 medium-sized orange, chopped

½ cup of fresh cranberries

1 cup of Romaine lettuce, chopped

3 tbsp of lemon juice, freshly squeezed

¼ tsp of cinnamon, ground

1 tbsp of honey, raw

Preparation:

Wash the strawberries and cut into bite-sized pieces. Set aside.

Place the cranberries in a colander and wash under cold running water. Slightly drain and set aside.

Wash the lettuce thoroughly and roughly chop it. Set aside.

Peel the orange and divide into wedges. Cut each wedge in half and set aside.

In a small bowl, combine lemon juice, cinnamon, and honey. Stir until combined and set aside.

Now, combine strawberries, cranberries, and lettuce in a salad bowl. Drizzle with previously prepared dressing and serve immediately.

Nutrition information per serving: Kcal: 221, Protein: 2.9g, Carbs: 51.8g, Fats: 1.1g

48.   Scrambled Eggs with Broccoli

Ingredients:

1 cup of fresh broccoli, chopped

1 small onion, finely chopped

¼ cup of shallots, finely chopped

5 large eggs, beaten

2 tbsp of skim milk

1 tbsp of olive oil

1 tsp of salt

¼ tsp of Italian seasoning

Preparation:

Wash the broccoli under cold running water. Drain and cut into bite-sized pieces. Set aside.

In a medium bowl, whisk the eggs, milk, salt, and Italian seasoning.

Preheat the oil in a large frying pan over a medium-high temperature. Add onions and stir-fry for about 3-4 minutes, or until translucent. Add broccoli and cook for 5 minutes, or until tender. Pour the egg mixture and cook for about 2-3 minutes and then sprinkle with shallots. Cook for 2 more minutes and remove from the heat.

Serve immediately.

Nutrition information per serving: Kcal: 290, Protein: 18.4g, Carbs: 11.4g, Fats: 19.8g

49.   Cooked Salmon with Spinach

Ingredients:

1 lb of wild salmon filets, boneless

1 lb of fresh spinach, torn

4 tbsp of olive oil

2 garlic cloves, finely chopped

2 tbsp of lemon juice

1 tbsp of fresh rosemary, chopped

1 tsp of sea salt

¼ tsp of black pepper, ground

Preparation:

Wash the salmon under cold running water and pat dry with a kitchen paper. Set aside.

Wash the spinach thoroughly and drain. Cut into small pieces and set aside.

Grease the bottom of a deep pot with 2 tablespoons of olive oil. Place salmon fillets and season with rosemary, salt, and pepper. Drizzle with lemon juice, add about ½ cup of water and cover with a lid. Bring it to a boil and then reduce the heat to low. Cook for about 30-40 minutes and then remove from the heat. Set aside.

Meanwhile, preheat the oil in a large saucepan over a medium-high heat. Add garlic and stir-fry for 3 minutes. Add spinach and 1 cup of water. Bring it to a boil and cook for 5 minutes. Remove from the heat.

Serve the salmon with spinach. I'm a huge fan of olive oil and I like to sprinkle some more before serving, but this is totally optional.

Nutrition information per serving: Kcal: 432, Protein: 44.9g, Carbs: 2.1g, Fats: 28.3g

50. Okra Soup

Ingredients:

1 cup of okra, chopped

3.5 oz of carrots, finely chopped

3.5 oz of celery root, finely chopped

A handful of green peas, soaked

2 tbsp of butter

2 tbsp of fresh parsley, finely chopped

1 egg yolk

2 tbsp of kaymak cheese

¼ cup of lemon juice, freshly squeezed

1 bay leaf

1 tsp of salt

½ tsp of black pepper, ground

4 cups of beef broth

1 cup of water

Preparation:

Wash and prepare the vegetables.

Melt the butter in a deep pot over a medium-high temperature. Add chopped okra, carrots, and celery. Cook for 5 minutes, stirring occasionally. Sprinkle with salt and pepper to taste.

Now, add broth, water, and green peas. Bring it to a boil and then reduce the heat to low. Cook for 25-30 minutes and then stir in the cheese, lemon juice, bay leaf, and egg yolk. Cook for 5 more minutes and then remove from the heat.

Serve warm and enjoy!

Nutrition information per serving: Kcal: 166, Protein: 7.7g, Carbs: 11g, Fats: 10.1g

51.   Turkey with Green Peppers

Ingredients:

1 lb turkey breasts, skinless and boneless

4 large green bell peppers, finely chopped

2 large potatoes, peeled and finely chopped

2 small carrots, sliced

2 ½ cups of chicken broth

1 large tomato, roughly chopped

3 tbsp of olive oil

1 tbsp of cayenne pepper

1 tsp of chili pepper, ground

1 tsp of salt

Preparation:

Wash the turkey breasts under cold running water and pat dry with a kitchen paper. Set aside.

Wash the bell peppers and cut lengthwise in half. Remove the seeds and cut into bite-sized pieces.

Peel the potatoes and cut into small chunks. Set aside.

Wash the tomato and roughly chop it. Set aside.

Preheat the oil in a large skillet over a medium-high temperature. Add meat and cook for about 4-5 minutes on each side. Add peppers, tomato, carrots, and potatoes. Stir and cook for 2 minutes and then add broth. Bring it to a boil and then reduce the heat to low. Sprinkle with salt, cayenne, and chili. Stir well and cook for 45 minutes. Remove from the heat.

Sprinkle with fresh parsley before serving.

Nutrition information per serving: Kcal: 325, Protein: 11.5g, Carbs: 44.5g, Fats: 12.8g

52.   Lamb Ragout

Ingredients:

1 lb lamb chops, 1-inch thick

1 cup of green peas, rinsed

4 medium-sized carrots, peeled and finely chopped

3 small onions, peeled and finely chopped

1 large potato, peeled and finely chopped

1 large tomato, peeled and roughly chopped

3 tbsp of olive oil

1 tbsp of cayenne pepper

1 tsp of salt

½ tsp of black pepper, freshly ground

Preparation:

Rinse the lamb chops under cold running water and pat dry with a kitchen paper. Cut into bite-sized pieces and set aside.

Wash and peel the carrots, potato, tomato and onion. Cut the carrot into thin slices and place in a deep pot. Cut the potato into small chunks and add it to the pot. Peel the onion and finely chop it.

Preheat the oil in a heavy bottomed pot over a medium-high temperature. Add meat chops and cook for 10 minutes, stirring occasionally.

Now, add all vegetables and stir well. Sprinkle with cayenne pepper, salt, and pepper to taste and give it a good stir. Add one cup of water and bring it to a boil. Reduce the heat to low and cook for 1 hour.

Remove from the heat and serve warm.

Nutrition information per serving: Kcal: 307, Protein: 24.9g, Carbs: 23.3g, Fats: 13g

53. Trout with Spinach and Potatoes

Ingredients:

2 medium-sized trout, cleaned

1 cup of fresh spinach, torn

2 large potatoes, peeled and sliced

3 garlic cloves, crushed

1 cup of olive oil

1 tsp of dried rosemary, finely chopped

2 springs of fresh mint leaves, chopped

1 lemon, juiced

1 tsp of sea salt

Preparation:

Wash the fish thoroughly under cold running water. Open the belly and wash inside as well. Pat dry with a kitchen paper and set aside.

Wash the spinach thoroughly and torn it. Set aside.

In a large bowl, combine olive oil, garlic, rosemary, mint, lemon juice, and salt. Stir until well incorporated. Place the fish in this marinade and wrap the bowl with a plastic foil. Refrigerate for 1 hour before grilling.

Meanwhile, place the spinach in a pot of boiling water. Cook for 3 minutes and remove from the heat. Drain well and set aside.

Place the potatoes in a pot of boiling water and cook for 10 minutes. Remove from the heat and drain well. Set aside.

Preheat the grill to a medium-high temperature. Place the fish and grill for about 5-7 minutes on each side. Brush the fish with remaining marinade while grilling.

Remove from the grill spinach and potatoes. Drizzle all with the remaining marinade and serve with some lemon wedges.

Enjoy!

Nutrition information per serving: Kcal: 318, Protein: 20.3g, Carbs: 31.9g, Fats: 12.6g

54.   Slow-Cooked White Peas

Ingredients:

1 lb of white peas

4 slices of bacon

1 large onion, finely chopped

1 small chili pepper, finely chopped

2 tbsp of all-purpose flour

2 tbsp of butter

1 tbsp of cayenne pepper

3 bay leaves, dried

1 tsp of salt

½ tsp of freshly ground black pepper

Preparation:

Melt 2 tablespoons of butter in a slow cooker. Add chopped onion and stir well. Now add bacon, peas, finely chopped chili pepper, bay leaves, salt, and pepper. Gently stir in 2 tablespoons of flour and add 3 cups of water.

Securely close the lid and cook for 8-9 hours on low setting or 5 hours on high setting.

Nutrition information per serving: Kcal: 210, Protein: 4g, Carbs: 24g, Fats: 12g

55.   Chickpea Pepper Soup

Ingredients:

14 oz chickpeas, soaked

2 large red bell peppers, finely chopped

2 small onions, peeled and finely chopped

2 large tomatoes, peeled and finely chopped

3 tbsp of tomato paste

A handful of fresh parsley, finely chopped

2 cups of vegetable broth

3 tbsp of extra virgin olive oil

1 tsp of salt

Preparation:

Soak the chickpeas overnight. Rinse and drain. Place the chickpeas in a pot of boiling water and cook for 30 minutes. Remove from the heat and drain. Set aside.

Wash the bell pepper and cut lengthwise in half. remove the seeds and finely chop it. Set aside.

Preheat the oil in a large saucepan over a medium-high temperature. Add onions and bell peppers. Cook for 5 minutes, or until tender. Add tomatoes, tomato paste, and parsley. Stir well and cook for 2 minutes. Now, add chickpeas and broth. Sprinkle with salt and stir again. Bring it to a boil and reduce the heat to low. Cook for 30 minutes and remove from the heat.

Serve warm.

Nutrition information per serving: Kcal: 424, Protein: 19.1g, Carbs: 59.4g, Fats: 14.1g

ADDITIONAL TITLES FROM THIS AUTHOR

70 Effective Meal Recipes to Prevent and Solve Being Overweight: Burn Fat Fast by Using Proper Dieting and Smart Nutrition

By

Joe Correa CSN

48 Acne Solving Meal Recipes: The Fast and Natural Path to Fixing Your Acne Problems in Less Than 10 Days!

By

Joe Correa CSN

41 Alzheimer's Preventing Meal Recipes: Reduce or Eliminate Your Alzheimer's Condition in 30 Days or Less!

By

Joe Correa CSN

70 Effective Breast Cancer Meal Recipes: Prevent and Fight Breast Cancer with Smart Nutrition and Powerful Foods

By

Joe Correa CSN

www.ingramcontent.com/pod-product-compliance
Lightning Source LLC
Chambersburg PA
CBHW030250030426
42336CB00009B/327